Dash Diet Recipes Book

50 Flavorful and Balanced Recipes for Your Healthy Everyday Meals

Natalie Puckett

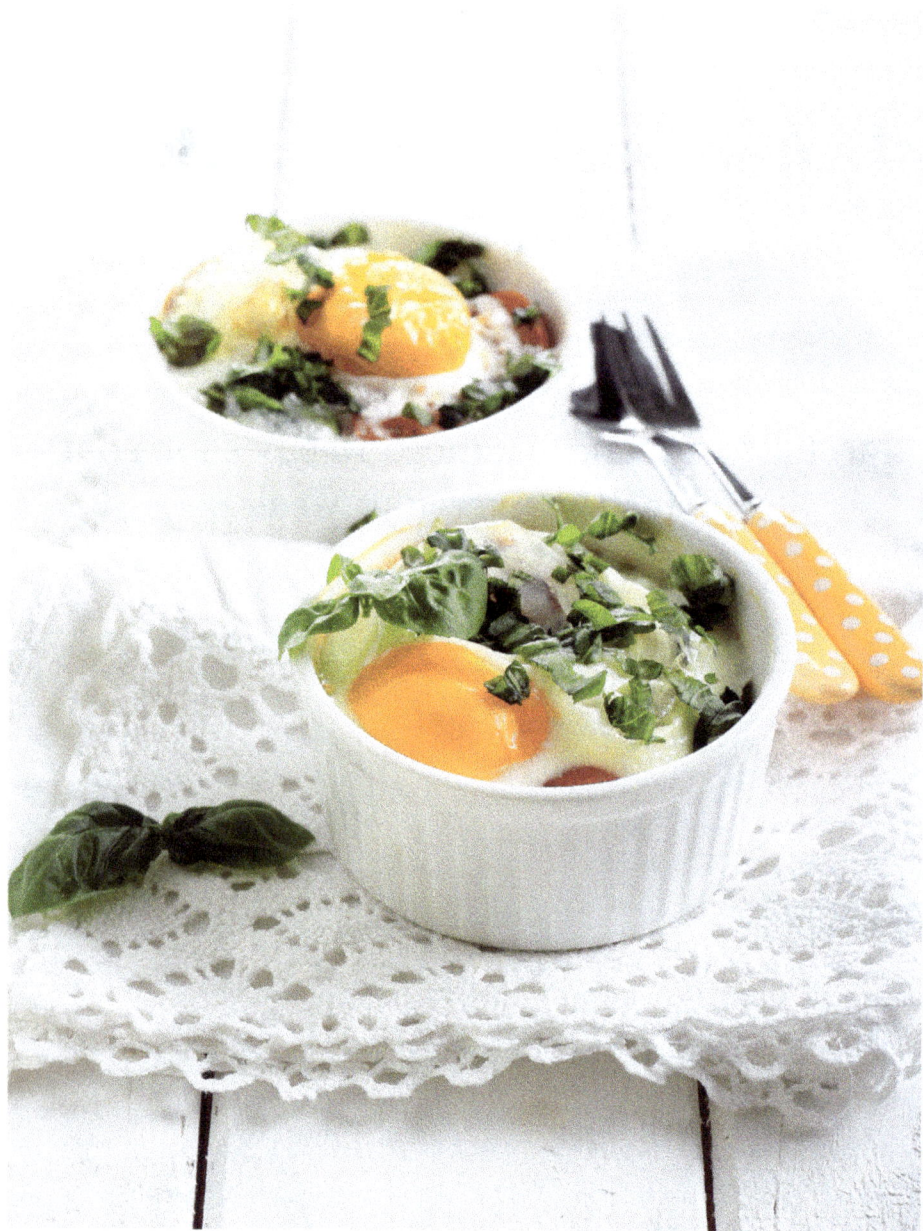

Table of Contents

Basil and Tomato Baked Eggs

Serving: 2

Prep Time: 10 minutes

Cook Time: 15 minutes

Ingredients:

1/2 garlic clove, minced

1/2 cup canned tomatoes

¼ cup fresh basil leaves, roughly chopped 1/4 teaspoon chili powder 1/2 tablespoon olive oil

2 whole eggs

Pepper to taste

How To:

1.   Preheat your oven to 375 degrees F.

2.   Take alittle baking dish and grease with vegetable oil .

3.   Add garlic, basil, tomatoes chili, vegetable oil into a dish and stir.

4.   Crack eggs into a dish, keeping space between the 2 .

5. Sprinkle the entire dish with sunflower seeds and pepper.

6. Place in oven and cook for 12 minutes until eggs are set and tomatoes are bubbling.

7. Serve with basil on top.

Enjoy!

Nutrition (Per Serving)

Calories: 235

Fat: 16g

Carbohydrates: 7g

Protein: 14g

Spanish Mussels

Serving: 4

Prep Time: 10 minutes

Cook Time: 23 minutes

Ingredients:

tablespoons olive oil

pounds mussels, scrubbed

Pepper to taste

cups canned tomatoes, crushed

shallot, chopped

garlic cloves, minced

cups low sodium vegetable stock

1/3 cup cilantro, chopped

How To:

1.   Take a pan and place it over medium-high heat, add shallot and stir-cook for 3 minutes.

2.   Add garlic, stock, tomatoes, pepper, stir and reduce heat, simmer for 10 minutes.

3.   Add mussels, cilantro, and toss.

4.   Cover and cook for 10 minutes more.

5.   Serve and enjoy!

Nutrition (Per Serving)

Calories: 210

Fat: 2g

Carbohydrates: 5g

Protein: 8g

Tilapia Broccoli Platter

Serving: 2

Prep Time: 4 minutes

Cook Time: 14 minutes

Ingredients:

Ounce tilapia, frozen

1 tablespoon almond butter

1 tablespoon garlic, minced

1 teaspoon lemon pepper seasoning

1 cup broccoli florets, fresh

How To:

1.   Pre-heat your oven to 350 degrees F.

2.   Add fish in aluminum foil packets.

3.   Arrange broccoli around fish.

4.   Sprinkle lemon pepper on top.

5.   Close the packets and seal.

6.   Bake for 14 minutes.

7.   Take a bowl and add garlic and almond butter, mix well and keep the mixture on the side.

8.   Remove the packet from oven and transfer to platter.

9.   Place almond butter on top of the fish and broccoli, serve and enjoy!

Nutrition (Per Serving)

Calories: 362

Fat: 25g

Carbohydrates: 2g

Protein: 29g

Salmon with Peas and Parsley Dressing

Serving: 4

Prep Time: 15 minutes

Cook Time: 15 minutes

Ingredients:

16 ounces salmon fillets, boneless and skin-on

1 tablespoon parsley, chopped

10 ounces peas

9 ounces vegetable stock, low sodium

2 cups water

½ teaspoon oregano, dried

½ teaspoon sweet paprika

2 garlic cloves, minced

A pinch of black pepper

How To:

1.   Add garlic, parsley, paprika, oregano and stock to a kitchen appliance and blend.

2.   Add water to your Pressure Pot.

3.   Add steam basket.

4.   Add fish fillets inside the steamer basket.

5.   Season with pepper.

6.   Lock the lid and cook on high for 10 minutes.

7.   Release the pressure naturally over 10 minutes .

8.   Divide the fish amongst plates.

9.   Add peas to the steamer basket and lock the lid again, cook on high for five minutes.

10.   Quick release the pressure.

11.   Divide the peas next to your fillets and serve with the parsley dressing drizzled

12.   on top

13.   Enjoy!

Nutrition (Per Serving)

Calories: 315

Fat: 5g

Carbohydrates: 14g

Protein: 16g

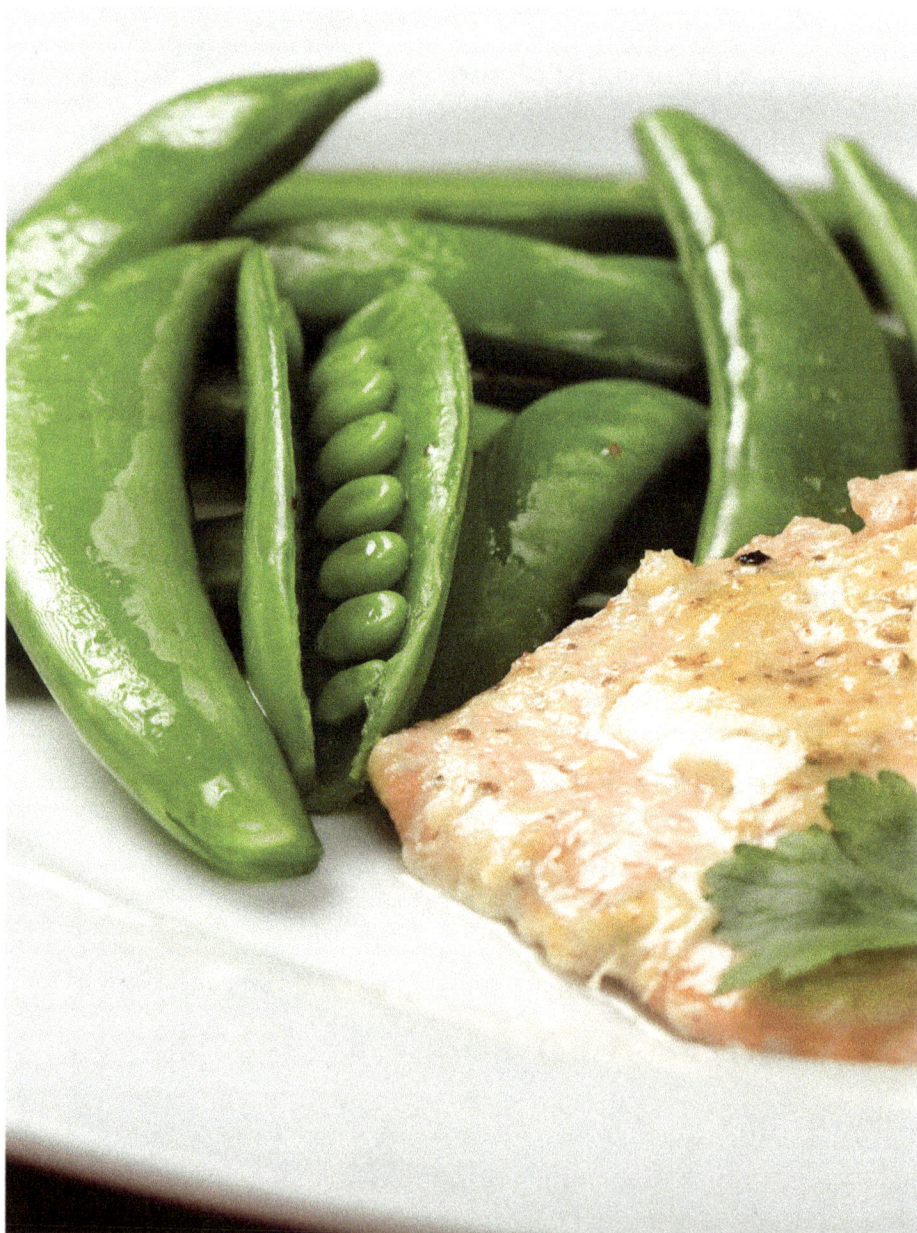

Mackerel and Orange Medley

Serving: 4

Prep Time: 10 minutes

Cook Time: 10 minutes

Ingredients:

mackerel fillets, skinless and boneless

spring onion, chopped

1 teaspoon olive oil

1-inch ginger piece, grated

Black pepper as needed

Juice and zest of 1 whole orange

1 cup low sodium fish stock

How To:

1.   Season the fillets with black pepper and rub vegetable oil .

2.   Add stock, fruit juice , ginger, orange peel and onion to Pressure Pot.

3.   Place a steamer basket and add the fillets.

4.   Lock the lid and cook on high for 10 minutes.

5.   Release the pressure naturally over 10 minutes.

6.   Divide the fillets amongst plates and drizzle the orange sauce from the pot over the fish.

7.   Enjoy!

Nutrition (Per Serving)

Calories: 200

Fat: 4g

Carbohydrates: 19g

Protein: 14g

Spicy Chili Salmon

Serving: 4

Prep Time: 10 minutes

Cook Time: 7 minutes

Ingredients:

salmon fillets, boneless and skin-on

2 tablespoons assorted chili peppers, chopped Juice of 1 lemon

1 lemon, sliced

1 cup water

Black pepper

How To:

1.   Add water to the moment Pot.

2.   Add steamer basket and add salmon fillets, season the fillets with salt and pepper.

3.   Drizzle juice on top.

4.   Top with lemon slices.

5.   Lock the lid and cook on high for 7 minutes.

6.   Release the pressure naturally over 10 minutes.

7.   Divide the salmon and lemon slices between serving plates.

8.   Enjoy!

Nutrition (Per Serving)

Calories: 281

Fats: 8g

Carbs: 19g

Protein:7g

Niçoise Salad with Tuna Steak

Nutrition

Calories: 956 kcal | Gross carbohydrates: 6 g | Protein: 37 g |
Fats: 86 g |Fiber: 2 g | Net carbohydrates: 4 g | Macro fats: 68 %
| Macro proteins: 29 % |Macro carbohydrates: 3 %

Total time: 18 minutes

Ingredients

Tuna steaks

375 grams of tuna steaks If you use frozen food, defrost
beforehand.

3 tablespoons butter

Eggs

3 eggs

Vegetable

0.5 celeriac

90 grams of cherry tomatoes

180-gram haricot verts Drained weight - from a pot without
added sugar

1 bunch of radishes

1 tablespoon capers

3 tablespoons olives If you buy olives in oil, make sure they are in olive oil and not in any other type of oil!

Dressing

300 ml mayonnaise

Instructions

1. Eggs

2. Start by boiling the eggs. Cook them in 8 minutes and then put them in a pan with cold water to cool.

3. Peel and halve the eggs.

4. Place the eggs on a large flat dish.

5. Tuna steaks

6. Melt the butter or ghee in a skillet or use a grill pan without butter.

7. Cook the tuna in 2.5 minutes per side (or until cooked, depending on the thickness of the tuna steak).

8. Place the tuna steaks on top of the haricot verts.

9. Vegetable

10. Use half a celery tuber. Cut the half tuber into 1.5 cm thick slices. Remove the skin and cut the slices into small cubes (approximately 1 cm -1.5 cm). Cook the cubes in the microwave or in a saucepan with some water. Allow to cool.

11. Drain the haricot verts and then place them in the middle of the serving dish. Still have room for the celery tuber.

12. Wash the tomatoes and halve them. Arrange them on the edge of the serving dish.

13. Wash the radishes and halve them. Place them on the edge of the serving dish.

14. Also, place the drained capers and olives on the edge of the serving dish.

15. Arrange the celery tuber cubes next to the haricot verts.

16. Sprinkle salt and pepper to taste over the eggs, tuna, and vegetables.

17. Serve with mayonnaise or mix in the mayonnaise.

Whole Grain Pasta with Meat Sauce

Prep time: 10 minutes

Cook time: 30 minutes

Servings: 6

Ingredients

Whole-grain pasta – 1 pound

Extra-lean ground beef – 1 pound

Onion – 1, diced

Garlic – 3 cloves, minced

No-salt-added tomato sauce – 2 (8-ounce) cans

Red wine – 1/3 cup

Balsamic vinegar – 1 Tbsp.

Dried basil - 1 tsp.

Dried marjoram – ½ tsp.

Dried oregano – ½ tsp.

Dried red pepper flakes - ½ tsp.

Dried thyme - ½ tsp.

Freshly ground black pepper - ½ tsp.

Method

1.   Follow the direction on the package and cook the pasta. Omit the salt. Drain and set aside.

2.   Place onion, ground beef and garlic in a pan over medium heat. Stir-fry for 5 minutes, or until the beef has browned.

3.   Add remaining ingredients and stir to combine. Simmer, uncovered, for 10 minutes, stirring occasionally.

4.   Remove from heat and spoon over pasta.

5.   Serve.

Nutritional Facts Per Serving

Calories: 387

Fat: 5g

Carb: 58g

Protein: 27g

Sodium 65mg

Beef Tacos

Prep time: 10 minutes

Cook time: 20 minutes

Servings: 6

Ingredients

Extra-lean ground beef – 1 pound

Large onion – 1, chopped Garlic – 2 cloves, minced

No-salt-added tomato sauce – 1 (8-ounce) can Low-sodium

Worcestershire sauce – 2 tsp.

Molasses - 1 Tbsp.

Apple cider vinegar – 1 Tbsp.

Ground cumin – 1 Tbsp.

Ground sweet paprika – 1 Tbsp.

Dried red pepper flakes - ½ tsp.

Ground black pepper to taste

Low-sodium taco shells – 1 package

Chopped fresh cilantro - ¼ cup Tomato and lettuce of serving

Method

1.   Place the ground beef, onion, and garlic in a pan over medium heat.

2.   Stir-fry for 5 minutes or until the beef is browned.

3.   Lower heat to medium-low and add the Worcestershire sauce, tomato sauce, molasses, vinegar, cumin, red pepper flakes, paprika, and black pepper. Simmer, stirring frequently, about 10 minutes.

4.   Heat taco shells according to package directions. Set aside.

5.   Remove the sauté pan from the heat. Stir in cilantro.

6.   Divide evenly between the taco shells.

7.   Garnish with lettuce, tomato and serve.

Nutritional Facts Per Serving (2 tacos)

Calories: 255

Fat: 9g

Carb: 23g

Protein: 18g

Sodium 79mg

Dirty Rice

Prep time: 10 minutes

Cook time: 30 minutes

Servings: 4

Ingredients

Extra-lean ground beef - ½ pound

Large onion – 1, diced

Celery – 2 stalks, diced

Garlic – 2 cloves, minced

Bell pepper – 1, diced

Sodium-free beef bouillon granules - 1 tsp.

Water - 1 cup

Low-sodium Worcestershire sauce – 2 tsp.

Dried thyme – 1 ½ tsp.

Dried basil – 1 tsp.

Dried marjoram - ½ tsp.

Ground black pepper - ¼ tsp.

Pinch ground cayenne pepper

Scallions – 2, diced

Cooked long-grain brown rice – 3 cups

Method

1.   In a pan, place the onion, ground beef, celery, and garlic. Stir-fry for 5 minutes or until beef is browned.

2.   Add beef bouillon, bell pepper, water, sauce, and herbs and stir to combine.

3.   Bring to a boil.

4.   Then reduce heat to low, and cover.

5.   Simmer for 20 minutes.

6.   Stir in the scallions and simmer, uncovered, for 3 minutes.

7.   Remove from heat. Add cooked rice and stir to combine.

8.   Serve.

Nutritional Facts Per Serving

Calories: 272

Fat: 4g

Carb: 41g

Protein: 16g

Sodium 92mg

Healthy Berry Cobbler

Serving: 8

Prep Time: 10 minutes

Cooking Time: 2 hours 30 minutes

Ingredients:

1 ¼ cups almond flour

1 cup coconut sugar

1 teaspoon baking powder

½ teaspoon cinnamon powder

1 whole egg

¼ cup low-fat milk

2 tablespoons olive oil

2 cups raspberries

2 cups blueberries

How To:

1.   Take a bowl and add almond flour, coconut sugar, baking powder and cinnamon.

2.   Stir well.

3.   Take another bowl and add egg, milk, oil, raspberries, blueberries and stir.

4.   Combine both of the mixtures.

5.   Grease your Slow Cooker.

6.   Pour the combined mixture into your Slow Cooker and cook on HIGH for 2 hours 30 minutes.

7.   Divide between serving bowls and enjoy!

Nutrition (Per Serving)

Calories: 250

Fat: 4g

Carbohydrates: 30g

Protein: 3g

Tasty Poached Apples

Serving: 8

Prep Time: 10 minutes

Cooking Time: 2 hours 30 minutes

Ingredients:

6 apples, cored, peeled and sliced

1 cup apple juice, natural

1 cup coconut sugar

1 tablespoon cinnamon powder

How To:

1. Grease Slow Cooker with cooking spray.

2. Add apples, sugar, juice, cinnamon to your Slow Cooker.

3. Stir gently.

4. Place lid and cook on HIGH for 4 hours.

5. Serve cold and enjoy!

Nutrition (Per Serving)

Calories: 180

Fat: 5g

Carbohydrates: 8g

Protein: 4g

Home Made Mix for The Trip

Serving: 4

Prep Time: 10 minutes

Cook Time: 55 minutes

Ingredients:

¼ cup raw cashews

¼ cup almonds

¼ cup walnuts

1 teaspoon cinnamon

2 tablespoons melted coconut oil

Sunflower seeds as needed

How To:

1.   Line baking sheet with parchment paper.

2.   Pre-heat your oven to 275 degrees F.

3.   Melt coconut oil and keep it on the side.

4.   Combine nuts to large mixing bowl and add cinnamon and melted coconut oil.

5.   Stir.

6.   Sprinkle sunflower seeds.

7.   Place in oven and brown for 6 minutes.

8.   Enjoy!

Nutrition (Per Serving)

Calories: 363

Fat: 22g

Carbohydrates: 41g

Protein: 7g

Heart Warming Cinnamon Rice Pudding

Serving: 4

Prep Time: 10 minutes

Cooking Time: 5 hours

Ingredients:

6 ½ cups water

1 cup coconut sugar

2 cups white rice

2 cinnamon sticks

½ cup coconut, shredded

How To:

1.   Add water, rice, sugar, cinnamon and coconut to your Slow Cooker.

2.   Gently stir.

3.   Place lid and cook on HIGH for 5 hours.

4.   Discard cinnamon.

5.   Divide pudding between dessert dishes and enjoy!

Nutrition (Per Serving)

Calories: 173

Fat: 4g

Carbohydrates: 9g

Protein: 4g

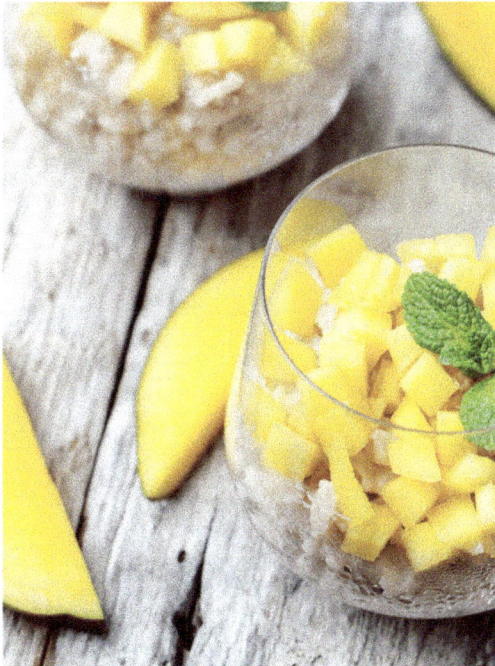

Pure Avocado Pudding

Serving: 4

Prep Time: 3 hours

Cook Time: nil

Ingredients:

1 cup almond milk

2 avocados, peeled and pitted

¾ cup cocoa powder

1 teaspoon vanilla extract

2 tablespoons stevia

¼ teaspoon cinnamon

Walnuts, chopped for serving

How To:

1.   Add avocados to a blender and pulse well.

2.   Add cocoa powder, almond milk, stevia, vanilla bean extract and pulse the mixture well.

3.   Pour into serving bowls and top with walnuts.

4. Chill for 2-3 hours and serve!

Nutrition (Per Serving)

Calories: 221

Fat: 8g

Carbohydrates: 7g

Protein: 3g

Sweet Almond and Coconut Fat Bombs

Serving: 6

Prep Time: 10 minutes

Cooking Time: 10 minutes

Freeze Time: 20 minutes

Ingredients:

¼ cup melted coconut oil

9 ½ tablespoons almond butter

90 drops liquid stevia

3 tablespoons cocoa

9 tablespoons melted almond butter, sunflower seeds

How To:

1.   Take a bowl and add all of the listed ingredients.

2.   Mix them well.

3.   Pour 2 tablespoons of the mixture into as many muffin molds as you like.

4.   Chill for 20 minutes and pop them out.

5.   Serve and enjoy!

Nutrition (Per Serving)

Total Carbs: 2g

Fiber: 0g

Protein: 2.53g

Fat: 14g

Spicy Popper Mug Cake

Serving: 2

Prep Time: 5 minutes

Cook Time: 5 minutes

Ingredients:

2 tablespoons almond flour

1 tablespoon flaxseed meal

1 tablespoon almond butter

1 tablespoon cream cheese

1 large egg

1 bacon, cooked and sliced

½ jalapeno pepper

½ teaspoon baking powder

¼ teaspoon sunflower seeds

How To:

1.   Take a frying pan and place it over medium heat.

2.   Add slice of bacon and cook until it has a crispy texture.

3. Take a microwave proof container and mix all of the listed ingredients (including cooked bacon), clean the sides.

4. Microwave for 75 seconds, making to put your microwave to high power.

5. Take out the cup and tap it against a surface to take the cake out.

6. Garnish with a bit of jalapeno and serve!

Nutrition (Per Serving)

Calories: 429

Fat: 38g

Carbohydrates: 6g

Protein: 16g

Sensational Strawberry Medley

Serving: 2

Prep Time: 5 minutes

Ingredients:

1-2 handful baby greens

3 medium kale leaves

5-8 mint leaves

1-inch piece ginger , peeled

1 avocado

1 cup strawberries

6-8 ounces coconut water + 6-8 ounces filtered water Fresh juice of one lime

1-2 teaspoon olive oil

How To:

1.   Add all the listed ingredients to your blender.

2.   Blend until smooth.

3.   Add a few ice cubes and serve the smoothie.

4.   Enjoy!

Nutrition (Per Serving)

Calories: 200

Fat: 10g

Carbohydrates: 14g

Protein 2g

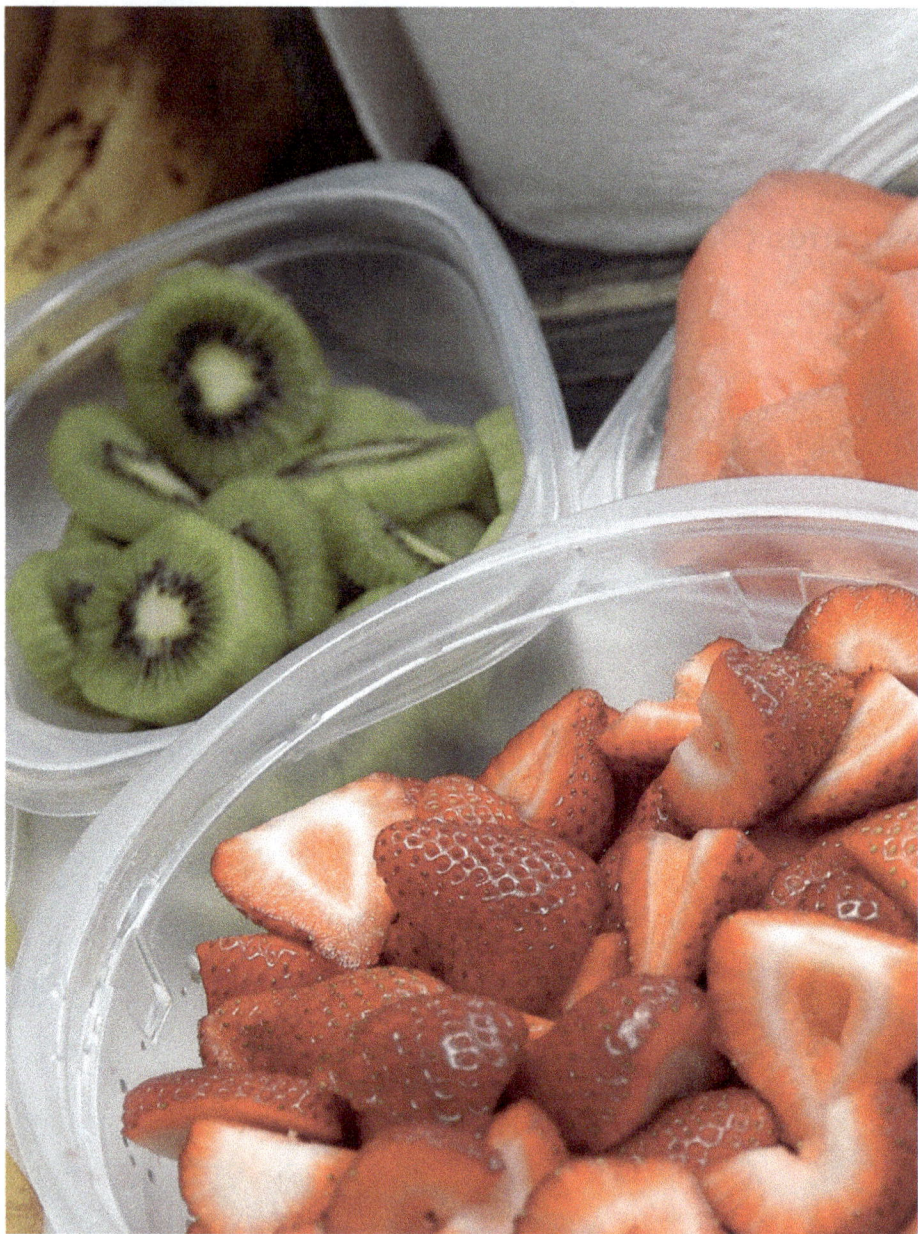

Mango's Gone Haywire

Serving: 2

Prep Time: 5 minutes

Ingredients:

1 mango, diced

2 bananas, diced

1-2 oranges, quartered

Dash of lemon juice

1 tablespoon hemp seed

¼ teaspoon green powder

Coconut water (as needed)

How To:

1.   Add orange quarters in the blender first, blend.

2.   Add the remaining ingredients and blend until smooth.

3.   Add more coconut water to adjust the thickness.

4.   Serve chilled!

Nutrition (Per Serving)

Calories: 200

Fat: 10g

Carbohydrates: 14g

Protein 2g

Unexpectedly Awesome Orange Smoothie

Serving: 2

Prep Time: 5 minutes

Ingredients:

1 orange, peeled

¼ cup fat-free yogurt

2 tablespoons frozen orange juice concentrate ¼ teaspoon vanilla extract

4 ice cubes

How To:

1.   Add the listed ingredients to your blender and blend until smooth.

2.   Serve chilled!

Nutrition (Per Serving)

Calories: 200

Fat: 10g

Carbohydrates: 14g

Protein 2g

Minty Cherry Smoothie

Serving: 2

Prep Time: 5 minutes

Ingredients:

¾ cup cherries

1 teaspoon mint

½ cup almond milk

½ cup kale

½ teaspoon fresh vanilla

How To:

1.   Wash and cut cherries.

2.   Take the pits out.

3.   Add cherries to blender.

4.   Pour almond milk.

5.   Wash the mint and put two sprigs in the blender.

6.   Separate the kale leaves from the stems.

7.   Put kale in blender.

8.   Press vanilla bean and cut lengthwise with knife.

9.   Scoop out your desired amount of vanilla and add to the blender.

10.   Blend until smooth.

11.   Serve chilled and enjoy!

Nutrition (Per Serving)

Calories: 200

Fat: 10g

Carbohydrates: 14g

Protein 2g

A Very Berry (and Green) Smoothie

Serving: 2

Prep Time: 5 minutes

Ingredients:

1 cup spinach leaves

½ cup frozen blueberries

1 ripe banana

½ cup milk

2 tablespoons old fashioned oats

½ tablespoon stevia

How To:

1.   Add the listed ingredients to your blender and blend until smooth.

2.   Serve chilled!

Nutrition (Per Serving)

Calories: 200

Fat: 10g

Carbohydrates: 14g

Protein 2g

Spicy Kale Chips

Serving: 4

Prep Time: 10 minutes

Cook Time: 25 minutes

Ingredients:

3 cups kale, stemmed and thoroughly washed, torn in 2-inch pieces

1 tablespoon extra-virgin olive oil

½ teaspoon chili powder

¼ teaspoon sea sunflower seeds

How To:

1.   Pre-heat your oven to 300 degrees F.

2.   Line 2 baking sheets with parchment paper and keep it on the side.

3.   Dry kale entirely and transfer to a large bowl.

4.   Add olive oil and toss.

5.   Make sure each leaf is covered.

6.   Season kale with chili powder and sunflower seeds, toss again.

7.   Divide kale between baking sheets and spread into a single layer.

8.   Bake for 25 minutes until crispy.

9.   Cool the chips for 5 minutes and serve.

10. Enjoy!

Nutrition (Per Serving)

Calories: 56

Fat: 4g

Carbohydrates: 5g

Protein: 2g

Seemingly Easy Portobello Mushrooms

Serving: 4

Prep Time: 10 minutes

Cook Time: 10 minutes

Ingredients:

12 cherry tomatoes

2 ounces scallions

4 portabella mushrooms

4 ¼ ounces almond butter

Sunflower seeds and pepper to taste

How To:

1.   Take a large skillet and melt almond butter over medium heat.

2.   Add mushrooms and sauté for 3 minutes.

3.   Stir in cherry tomatoes and scallions.

4.   Sauté for 5 minutes. 5. Season accordingly.

5.   Sauté until veggies are tender.

6.   Enjoy!

Nutrition (Per Serving)

Calories: 154

Fat: 10g

Carbohydrates: 2g

Protein: 7g

The Garbanzo Bean Extravaganza

Serving: 5

Prep Time: 10 minutes

Cook Time: Nil

Ingredients:

1 can garbanzo beans, chickpeas

1 tablespoon olive oil

1 teaspoon sunflower seeds

1 teaspoon garlic powder

½ teaspoon paprika

How To:

1.   Pre-heat your oven to 375 degrees F.

2.   Line a baking sheet with a silicone baking mat.

3.   Drain and rinse garbanzo beans, pat garbanzo beans dry and put into a large bowl.

4.   Toss with olive oil, sunflower seeds, garlic powder, paprika and mix well.

5.   Spread over a baking sheet.

6.   Bake for 20 minutes.

7.   Turn chickpeas so they are roasted well.

8.   Place back in oven and bake for another 25 minutes at 375 degrees F.

9.   Let them cool and enjoy!

Nutrition (Per Serving)

Calories: 395

Fat: 7g

Carbohydrates: 52g

Protein: 35g

Classic Guacamole

Serving: 6

Prep Time: 15 minutes

Cook Time: Nil

Ingredients:

3 large ripe avocados

1 large red onion, peeled and diced

4 tablespoons freshly squeezed lime juice Sunflower seeds as needed

Freshly ground black pepper as needed Cayenne pepper as needed

How To:

1.   Halve the avocados and discard stone.

2.   Scoop flesh from 3 avocado halves and transfer to a large bowl.

3.   Mash using a fork.

4.   Add 2 tablespoons of lime juice and mix.

5.   Dice the remaining avocado flesh (remaining half) and transfer to another bowl.

6.   Add remaining juice and toss.

7.   Add diced flesh with the mashed flesh and mix.

8.   Add chopped onions and toss.

9.   Season with sunflower seeds, pepper and cayenne pepper.

10.   Serve and enjoy!

Nutrition (Per Serving)

Calories: 172

Fat: 15g

Carbohydrates: 11g

Protein: 2g

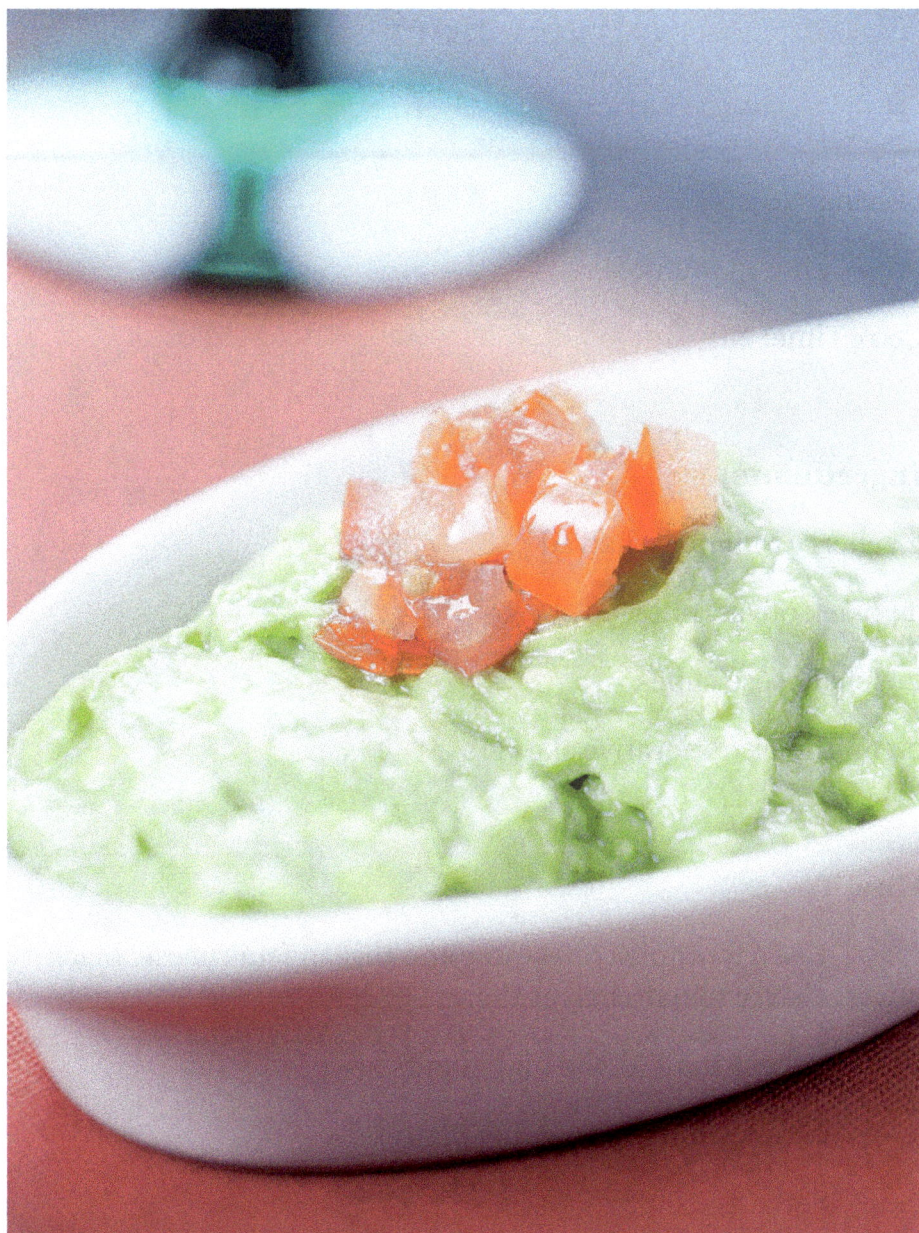

Olive Cherry Bites

Serving: 30

Prep Time: 15 minutes

Cook Time: Nil

Ingredients:

24 cherry tomatoes, halved

24 black olives, pitted

24 feta cheese cubes

24 toothpick/decorative skewers

How To:

1.   Use a toothpick or skewer and thread feta cheese, black olives, cherry tomato halves therein order.

2.   Repeat until all the ingredients are used.

3.   Arrange during a serving platter.

4.   Serve and enjoy!

Nutrition (Per Serving)

Calories: 57

Fat: 5g

Carbohydrates: 2g

Protein: 2g

Roasted Herb Crackers

Serving: 75 Crackers

Prep Time: 10 minutes

Cook Time: 120 minutes

Ingredients:

¼ cup avocado oil

10 celery sticks

1 sprig fresh rosemary, stem discarded

2 sprigs fresh thyme, stems discarded

2 tablespoons apple cider vinegar

1 teaspoon Himalayan sunflower seeds

3 cups ground flaxseeds

How To:

1.   Preheat your oven to 225 degrees F.

2.   Line a baking sheet with parchment paper and keep it on the side.

3.   Add oil, herbs, celery, vinegar, sunflower seeds to a kitchen appliance and pulse until you've got a good mixture.

4.   Add flax and puree.

5.   Let it sit for 2-3 minutes.

6.   Transfer batter to your prepared baking sheet and spread evenly, dig cracker shapes.

7.   Bake for hour , flip and bake for hour more.

8.   Enjoy!

Nutrition (Per Serving)

Calories: 34

Fat: 5g

Carbohydrates: 1g

Protein: 1.3g

Banana Steel Oats

Serving: 3

Prep Time: 10 minutes

Cook Time: 15 minutes

Ingredients:

1 small banana

1 cup almond milk

¼ teaspoon cinnamon, ground

½ cup rolled oats

1 tablespoon honey

How To:

1.   Take a saucepan and add half the banana, whisk in almond milk, ground cinnamon.

2.   Season with sunflower seeds.

3.   Stir until the banana is mashed well, bring the mixture to a boil and stir in oats.

4.   Reduce heat to medium-low and simmer for 5-7 minutes

until the oats are tender.

5. Dice the remaining half banana and placed on the highest of the oatmeal.

6. Enjoy!

Nutrition (Per Serving)

Calories: 358

Fat: 6g

Carbohydrates: 76g

Protein: 7g

Swiss Chard Omelet

Serving: 2

Prep Time: 5 minutes

Cook Time: 5 minutes

Ingredients:

2 eggs, lightly beaten

2 cups Swiss chard, sliced

1 tablespoon almond butter

½ teaspoon sunflower seeds Fresh pepper

How To:

1.   Take a non-stick frypan and place it over medium-low heat.

2.   Once the almond butter melts, add Swiss chard and stir-cook for two minutes.

3.   Pour the eggs into the pan and gently stir them into Swiss chard.

4.   Season with garlic sunflower seeds and pepper.

5.   Cook for two minutes.

6.   Serve and enjoy!

Nutrition (Per Serving)

Calories: 260

Fat: 21g

Carbohydrates: 4g

Protein: 14g

Hearty Pineapple Oatmeal

Serving: 5

Prep Time: 10 minutes

Cook Time: 4-8 hours

Ingredients:

1 cup steel-cut oats

4 cups unsweetened almond milk

2 medium apples, sliced

1 teaspoon coconut oil

1 teaspoon cinnamon

¼ teaspoon nutmeg

2 tablespoons maple syrup, unsweetened A drizzle of lemon juice

How To:

1.   Add listed ingredients to a pan and blend well.

2.   Cook on very low flame for 8 hours/or on high flame for 4 hours.

3.   Gently stir.

4.   Add your required toppings.

5.   Serve and enjoy!

6.   Store within the fridge for later use; confirm to feature a splash of almond milk after re-heating for added flavor.

Nutrition (Per Serving)

Calories: 180

Fat: 5g

Carbohydrates: 31g

Protein: 5g

Zingy Onion and Thyme Crackers

Serving: 75 crackers

Prep Time: 15 minutes

Cooking Time: 120 minutes

Ingredients:

1 garlic clove, minced

1 cup sweet onion, coarsely chopped

2 teaspoons fresh thyme leaves

¼ cup avocado oil

¼ teaspoon garlic powder

Freshly ground black pepper

¼ cup sunflower seeds

1 ½ cups roughly ground flax seeds

How To:

1.   Preheat your oven to 225 degrees F.

2.   Line two baking sheets with parchment paper and keep it on the side.

3.   Add garlic, onion, thyme, oil, sunflower seeds, and pepper to a kitchen appliance.

4.   Add sunflower and flax seeds, pulse until pureed.

5.   Transfer the batter to prepared baking sheets and spread evenly, dig crackers

6.   Bake for hour.

7.   Remove parchment paper and flip crackers, bake for an additional hour.

8.   If crackers are thick, it'll take longer.

9.   Remove from oven and allow them to cool.

10.   Enjoy!

Nutrition (Per Serving)

Total Carbs: 0.8g

Fiber: 0.2g

Protein: 0.4g

Fat: 2.7g

Crunchy Flax and Almond Crackers

Serving: 20-24 crackers

Prep Time: 15 minutes

Cooking Time: 60 minutes

Ingredients:

½ cup ground flaxseeds

½ cup almond flour

1 tablespoon coconut flour

2 tablespoons shelled hemp seeds

¼ teaspoon sunflower seeds

1 egg white

2 tablespoons unsalted almond butter, melted

How To:

1.   Preheat your oven to 300 degrees F.

2.   Line a baking sheet with parchment paper, keep it on the side.

3.   Add flax, almond, coconut flour, hemp seed, seeds to a bowl and blend.

4.   Add albumen and melted almond butter, mix until combined.

5.   Transfer dough to a sheet of parchment paper and canopy with another sheet of paper.

6.   Roll out dough.

7.   dig crackers and bake for hour.

8.   allow them to cool and enjoy!

Nutrition (Per Serving)

Total Carbs: 1.2

Fiber: 1g

Protein: 2g

Fat: 6g

Duck with Cucumber and Carrots

Serving: 8

Prep Time: 10 minutes

Cook Time: 40 minutes

Ingredients:

1 duck, cut up into medium pieces

1 chopped cucumber, chopped

1 tablespoon low sodium vegetable stock

2 carrots, chopped

2 cups of water

Black pepper as needed

1-inch ginger piece, grated

How To:

1.   Add duck pieces to your Pressure Pot.

2.   Add cucumber, stock, carrots, water, ginger, pepper and stir.

3.   Lock up the lid and cook on low for 40 minutes.

4.   Release the pressure naturally.

5.   Serve and enjoy!

Nutrition (Per Serving)

Calories: 206

Fats: 7g

Carbs: 28g

Protein: 16g

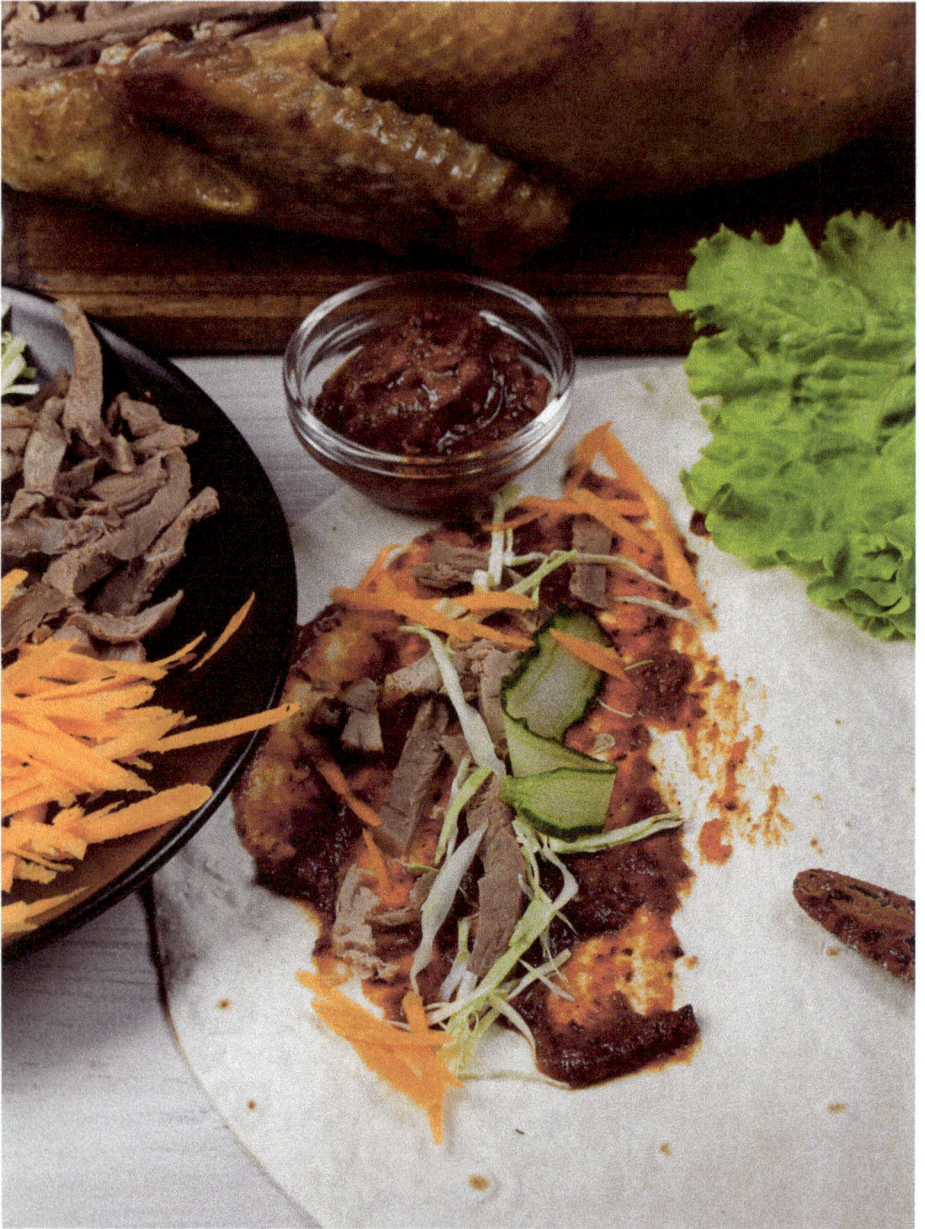

Parmesan Baked Chicken

Serving: 2

Prep Time: 5 minutes

Cook Time: 20 minutes

Ingredients:

2 tablespoons ghee

2 boneless chicken breasts, skinless

Pink sunflower seeds

Freshly ground black pepper

½ cup mayonnaise, low fat

¼ cup parmesan cheese, grated

1 tablespoon dried Italian seasoning, low fat, low sodium ¼ cup crushed pork rinds

How To:

1.   Preheat your oven to 425 degrees F.

2.   Take an outsized baking dish and coat with ghee.

3.   Pat chicken breasts dry and wrap with a towel.

4.   Season with sunflower seeds and pepper.

5.   Place in baking dish.

6.   Take a little bowl and add mayonnaise, parmesan cheese, Italian seasoning.

7.   Slather mayo mix evenly over pigeon breast.

8.   Sprinkle crushed pork rinds on top.

9.   Bake for 20 minutes until topping is browned.

10.   Serve and enjoy!

Nutrition (Per Serving)

Calories: 850

Fat: 67g

Carbohydrates: 2g

Protein: 60g

Buffalo Chicken Lettuce Wraps

Serving: 2

Prep Time: 35 minutes

Cook Time: 10 minutes

Ingredients:

3 chicken breasts, boneless and cubed

20 slices of almond butter lettuce leaves ¾ cup cherry tomatoes halved

1 avocado, chopped

¼ cup green onions, diced

½ cup ranch dressing

¾ cup hot sauce

How To:

1.   Take a bowl and add chicken cubes and sauce , mix.

2.   Place within the fridge and let it marinate for half-hour .

3.   Preheat your oven to 400 degrees F.

4. Place coated chicken on a cookie pan and bake for 9 minutes.

5. Assemble lettuce serving cups with equal amounts of lettuce, green onions, tomatoes, ranch dressing, and cubed chicken.

6. Serve and enjoy!

Nutrition (Per Serving)

Calories: 106

Fat: 6g

Net Carbohydrates: 2g

Protein: 5g

Crazy Japanese Potato and Beef Croquettes

Serving: 10

Prep Time: 10 minutes

Cook Time: 20 minutes

Ingredients:

3 medium russet potatoes, peeled and chopped

1 tablespoon almond butter

1 tablespoon vegetable oil

3 onions, diced

¾ pound ground beef

4 teaspoons light coconut aminos

All-purpose flour for coating

2 eggs, beaten

Panko bread crumbs for coating

½ cup oil, frying

How To:

1.   Take a saucepan and place it over medium-high heat; add potatoes and sunflower seeds water, boil for 16 minutes.

2.   Remove water and put potatoes in another bowl, add almond butter and mash the potatoes.

3.   Take a frypan and place it over medium heat, add 1 tablespoon oil and let it heat up.

4.   Add onions and fry until tender.

5.   Add coconut aminos to beef to onions.

6.   Keep frying until beef is browned.

7.   Mix the meat with the potatoes evenly.

8.   Take another frypan and place it over medium heat; add half a cup of oil.

9.   Form croquettes using the potato mixture and coat them with flour, then eggs and eventually breadcrumbs.

10.   Fry patties until golden on all sides.

11.   Enjoy!

Nutrition (Per Serving)

Calories: 239
Fat: 4g
Carbohydrates: 20g
Protein: 10g

Spicy Chili Crackers

Serving: 30 crackers

Prep Time: 15 minutes

Cooking Time: 60 minutes

Ingredients:

¾ cup almond flour

¼ cup coconut four

¼ cup coconut flour

½ teaspoon paprika

½ teaspoon cumin

1 ½ teaspoons chili pepper spice

1 teaspoon onion powder

½ teaspoon sunflower seeds

1 whole egg

¼ cup unsalted almond butter

How To:

1.   Preheat your oven to 350 degrees F.

2.   Line a baking sheet with parchment paper and keep it on the side.

3.   Add ingredients to your kitchen appliance and pulse until you've got a pleasant dough.

4.   Divide dough into two equal parts.

5.   Place one ball on a sheet of parchment paper and canopy with another sheet; roll it out.

6.   dig crackers and repeat with the opposite ball.

7.   Transfer the prepped dough to a baking tray and bake for 8-10 minutes.

8.   Remove from oven and serve.

9.   Enjoy!

Nutrition (Per Serving)

Total Carbs: 2.8g

Fiber: 1g

Protein: 1.6g

Fat: 4.1g

Zucchini Zoodles with Chicken and Basil

Serving: 2

Prep Time: 10 minutes

Cook Time: 10 minutes

Ingredients:

2 chicken fillets, cubed

2 tablespoons ghee

1-pound tomatoes, diced

½ cup basil, chopped

¼ cup coconut almond milk

1 garlic clove, peeled, minced

1 zucchini, shredded

How To:

1.   Sauté cubed chicken in ghee until not pink.

2.   Add tomatoes and season with sunflower seeds.

3.   Simmer and reduce the liquid.

4.   Prepare your zucchini Zoodles by shredding zucchini during a kitchen appliance.

5.   Add basil, garlic, coconut almond milk to chicken and cook for a couple of minutes.

6.   Add half the zucchini Zoodles to a bowl and top with creamy tomato basil chicken.

7.   Enjoy!

Nutrition (Per Serving)

Calories: 540

Fat: 27g

Carbohydrates: 13g

Protein: 59g

Tasty Roasted Broccoli

Serving: 4

Prep Time: 5 minutes

Cook Time: 20 minutes

Ingredients:

4 cups broccoli florets

1 tablespoon olive oil

Sunflower seeds and pepper to taste

How To:

1.   Pre-heat your oven to 400 degrees F.

2.   Add broccoli during a zip bag alongside oil and shake until coated.

3.   Add seasoning and shake again.

4.   Spread broccoli out on baking sheet, bake for 20 minutes.

5.   Let it cool and serve.

6.   Enjoy!

Nutrition (Per Serving)

Calories: 62

Fat: 4g

Carbohydrates: 4g

Protein: 4g

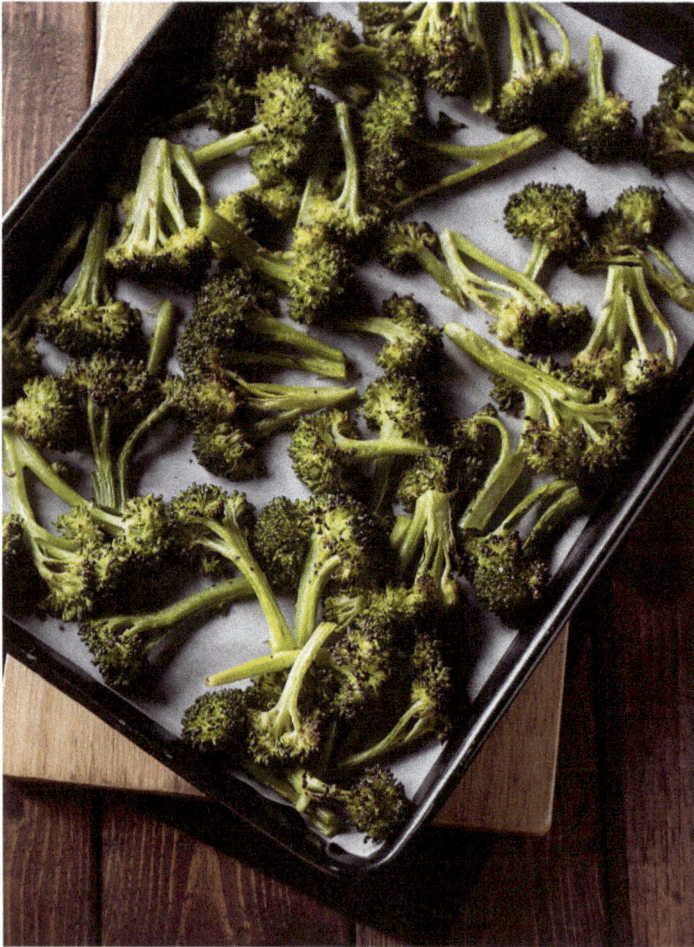

The Almond Breaded Chicken Goodness

Serving: 3

Prep Time: 15 minutes

Cook Time: 15 minutes

Ingredients:

2 large chicken breasts, boneless and skinless 1/3 cup lemon juice

1 ½ cups seasoned almond meal

2 tablespoons coconut oil

Lemon pepper, to taste

Parsley for decoration

How To:

1.   Slice pigeon breast in half.

2.   Pound out each half until ¼ inch thick.

3.   Take a pan and place it over medium heat, add oil and warmth it up.

4.   Dip each pigeon breast slice through juice and let it sit for two minutes.

5.   Turnover and therefore the let the opposite side sit for two minutes also.

6.   Transfer to almond meal and coat each side.

7.   Add coated chicken to the oil and fry for 4 minutes per side, ensuring to sprinkle lemon pepper liberally.

8.   Transfer to a paper lined sheet and repeat until all chicken are fried.

9.   Garnish with parsley and enjoy!

Nutrition (Per Serving)

Calories: 325

Fat: 24g

Carbohydrates: 3g

Protein: 16g

South-Western Pork Chops

Serving: 4

Prep Time: 10 minutes

Cook Time: 15 minutes

Smart Points: 3

Ingredients:

Cooking spray as needed 4-ounce pork loin chop, boneless and fat rimmed 1/3 cup salsa

2 tablespoons fresh lime juice

¼ cup fresh cilantro, chopped

How To:

1.   Take an outsized sized non-stick skillet and spray it with cooking spray.

2.   Heat until hot over high heat.

3.   Press the chops together with your palm to flatten them slightly.

4.   Add them to the skillet and cook on 1 minute for every side until they're nicely browned.

5.   Lower the warmth to medium-low.

6.   Combine the salsa and juice.

7.   Pour the combination over the chops.

8.   Simmer uncovered for about 8 minutes until the chops are perfectly done.

9.   If needed, sprinkle some cilantro on top.

10.   Serve!

Nutrition (Per Serving)

Calorie: 184

Fat: 4g

Carbohydrates: 4g

Protein: 0.5g

Ginger Zucchini Avocado Soup

Serving: 3

Prep Time: 7 minutes

Cook Time: 25 minutes

Ingredients:

1 red bell pepper, chopped

1 big avocado

1 teaspoon ginger, grated

Pepper as needed

2 tablespoons avocado oil

4 scallions, chopped

1 tablespoon lemon juice

29 ounces vegetable stock

1 garlic clove, minced

2 zucchini, chopped

1 cup water

How To:

1.   Take a pan and place over medium heat, add onion and fry for 3 minutes.

2.   Stir in ginger, garlic and cook for 1 minute.

3.   Mix in seasoning, zucchini stock, water and boil for 10 minutes.

4.   Remove soup from fire and let it sit, blend in avocado and blend using an immersion blender.

5.   Heat over low heat for a short time .

6.   Adjust your seasoning and add juice , bell pepper.

7.   Serve and enjoy!

Nutrition (Per Serving)

Calories: 155

Fat: 11g

Carbohydrates: 10g

Protein: 7g

Greek Lemon and Chicken Soup

Serving: 4

Prep Time: 15 minutes

Cook Time: 30 minutes

Ingredients:

2 cups cooked chicken, chopped

2 medium carrots, chopped

½ cup onion, chopped ¼ cup lemon juice 1 clove garlic, minced

1 can cream of chicken soup, fat-free and low sodium

2 cans chicken broth, fat-free

¼ teaspoon ground black pepper

2/3 cup long-grain rice

2 tablespoons parsley, snipped

How To:

1.   Add all of the listed ingredients to a pot (except rice and parsley).

2.   Season with sunflower seeds and pepper.

3. Bring the combination to a overboil medium-high heat.

4. Stir in rice and set heat to medium.

5. Simmer for 20 minutes until rice is tender.

6. Garnish parsley and enjoy!

Nutrition (Per Serving)

Calories: 582

Fat: 33g

Carbohydrates: 35g

Protein: 32g

Morning Peach

Serving: 4

Prep Time: 10 minutes

Cook Time: 5 minutes

Ingredients:

6 small peaches, cored and cut into wedges ¼ cup coconut sugar

2 tablespoons almond butter

¼ teaspoon almond extract

How To:

1.   Take alittle pan and add peaches, sugar, butter and flavor.

2.   Toss well.

3.   Cook over medium-high heat for five minutes, divide the combination into bowls and serve.

4.   Enjoy!

Nutrition (Per Serving)

Calories: 198

Fat: 2g

Carbohydrates: 11g

Protein: 8g

Garlic and Pumpkin Soup

Serving: 4

Prep Time: 10 minutes

Cook Time: 5 hours

Ingredients:

1-pound pumpkin chunks

1 onion, diced

2 cups vegetable stock

1 2/3 cups coconut cream

½ stick almond butter

1 teaspoon garlic, crushed

1 teaspoon ginger, crushed

Pepper to taste

How To:

1.   Add all the ingredients into your Slow Cooker.

2.   Cook for 4-6 hours on high.

3.   Puree the soup by using an immersion blender.

4.   Serve and enjoy!

Nutrition (Per Serving)

Calories: 235

Fat: 21g

Carbohydrates: 11g

Protein: 2g

Butternut and Garlic Soup

Serving: 4

Prep Time: 5 minutes

Cook Time: 35 minutes

Ingredients:

4 cups butternut squash, cubed

4 cups vegetable broth, stock

½ cup low fat cream

2 garlic cloves, chopped

Pepper to taste

How To:

1.   Add butternut squash, garlic cloves, broth, salt and pepper during a large pot.

2.   Place the pot over medium heat and canopy with the lid.

3.   Bring back boil then reduce the temperature.

4.   Let it simmer for 30-35 minutes.[MOU7]

5.   Blend the soup for 1-2 minutes until you get a smooth mixture.

6.   Stir the cream through the soup.

7.   Serve and enjoy!

Nutrition (Per Serving)

Calories: 180

Fat: 14g

Carbohydrates: 21g

Protein: 3g

Minty Avocado Soup

Serving: 4

Prep Time: 10 minutes + Chill time

Cook Time: nil

Ingredients:

1 avocado, ripe

1 cup coconut almond milk, chilled

2 romaine lettuce leaves

20 mint leaves, fresh

1 tablespoon lime juice

Sunflower seeds, to taste

How To:

1.   Activate your slow cooker and add all the ingredients into it.

2.   Mix them during a kitchen appliance.

3.   Make a smooth mixture.

4.   Let it chill for 10 minutes.

5. Serve and enjoy!

Nutrition (Per Serving)

Calories: 280

Fat: 26g

Carbohydrates: 12g

Protein: 4g

Celery, Cucumber and Zucchini Soup

Serving: 2

Prep Time: 10 minutes + Chill time

Cook Time: nil

Ingredients:

3 celery stalks, chopped

7 ounces cucumber, cubed

1 tablespoon olive oil

2/5 cup fresh cream, 30%, low fat

1 red bell pepper, chopped

1 tablespoon dill, chopped

10 ½ ounces zucchini, cubed

Sunflower seeds and pepper, to taste

How To:

1.   Put the vegetables during a juicer and juice.

2.   Then mix within the vegetable oil and fresh cream.

3.   Season with sauce and pepper.

4.   Garnish with dill.

5. Serve it chilled and enjoy!

Nutrition (Per Serving)

Calories: 325

Fat: 32g

Carbohydrates: 10g

Protein: 4g

Rosemary and Thyme Cucumber Soup

Serving: 3

Prep Time: 10 minutes + Chill time

Cook Time: nil

Ingredients:

4 cups vegetable broth

1 teaspoon thyme, freshly chopped

1 teaspoon rosemary, freshly chopped

2 cucumbers, sliced1 cup low fat cream

1 pinch of sunflower seeds

How To:

1.   Take an outsized bowl and add all the ingredients.

2.   Whisk well.

3.   Blend until smooth by using an immersion blender.

4.   Let it chill for 1 hour.

5.   Serve and enjoy!

Nutrition (Per Serving)

Calories: 111

Fat: 8g

Carbohydrates: 4g

Protein: 5g

Guacamole Soup

Serving: 3

Prep Time: 10 minute + Chill time

Cook Time: nil

Ingredients:

3 cups vegetable broth 2 ripe avocados, pitted ½ cup cilantro, freshly chopped

1 tomato, chopped

½ cup low fat cream

Sunflower seeds & black pepper, to taste

How To:

1.   Add all the ingredients into a blender.

2.   Blend until creamy by using an immersion blender.

3.   Let it chill for 1 hour.

4.   Serve and enjoy!

Nutrition (Per Serving)

Calories: 289

Fat: 26g

Carbohydrates: 5g

Protein: 10g

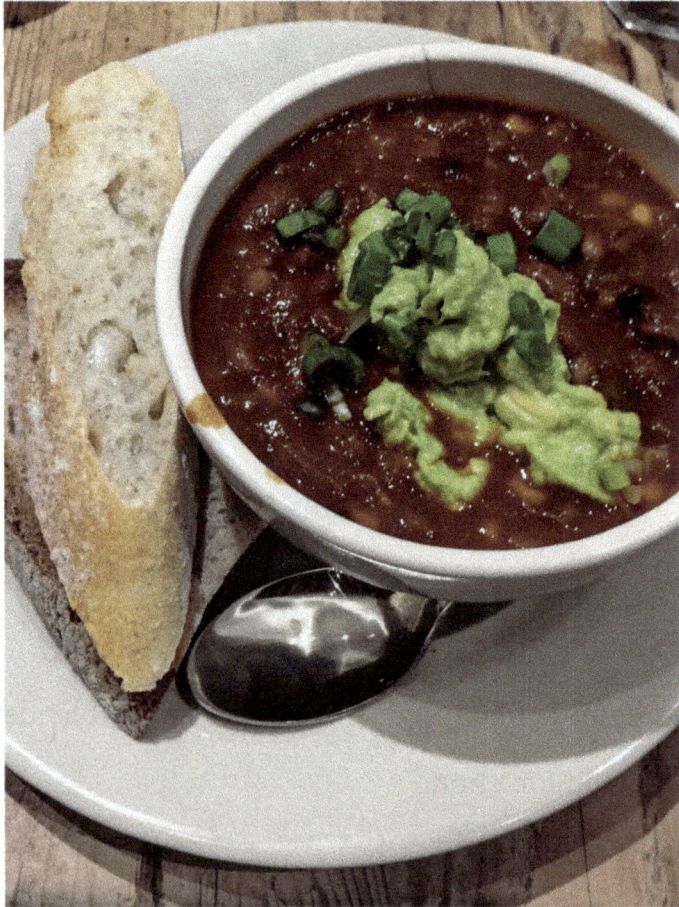